ALL YOU WANTED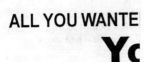
Yo

New Dawn B-62/14, Naraina Indl. Area Phase-II,
New Delhi-110 028. www.ubspd.com
ISBN 81-207-2232-X
Reprint 2001

LALITHA SHARMA

All rights reserved. No part of this publication may be reproduced, stored in a retrieval system, or transmitted in any form or by any means, electronic, mechanical, photocopying, recording and/or otherwise without the prior written permission of the publishers.

Printed at Saurabh Printers Pvt. Ltd., A-16, Sector-IV, NOIDA

New Dawn

NEW DAWN
An imprint of Sterling Publishers (P) Ltd.
L-10, Green Park Extension, New Delhi-110016
Ph.: 6191784, 6191785, 6191023 Fax: 91-11-6190028
E-mail: ghai@nde.vsnl.net.in
Internet: http://www.sterlingpublishers.com

All You Wanted To Know About — Yoga
©1999, Sterling Publishers Private Limited
ISBN 81 207 2232 9
Reprint 2001

All rights are reserved. No part of this publication may be
reproduced, stored in a retrieval system or transmitted, in any form
or by any means, mechanical, photocopying, recording or
otherwise, without prior written permission of the publisher.

Published by Sterling Publishers Pvt. Ltd., New Delhi-110016.
Lasertypeset by Vikas Compographics, New Delhi-110029.
Printed at Shagun Composer, New Delhi-110029.

Contents

Preface

This book is aimed at dealing with the physical aspect of Yoga, i.e. the Hatha Yoga. The carefully selected asanas, when practised, lead to a healthy long life. The practical illustrations prove very useful in the practice of the Yogic exercises. It is, however, very essential to seek the guidance of a master/instructor to attain perfection in the different postures.

Yoga surpasses any other method of improving the body viz. aerobics, jogging, athletics, and swimming, and reaches the emotional and mental aspects of a person and helps in bringing out inner beauty person.

The purpose of Yoga is to help eliminate tension, and to relax the body and mind. And once the body is aligned, tranquillity and serenity fills your being. Hatha Yoga builds strong legs, increases general vitality, improves blood circulation, coordination and balance. As the body and breath work in unison, one moves in a meditative state.

Introduction

The attitude towards Yoga and its acceptance has undergone a sea change over the last twenty years. This is true not only of our country where Yoga originated a thousand years ago, but also of far-flung countries all over the world.

Why has Yoga created such an awareness in the common person be he a business tycoon, professional, worker, housewife, student or child?

Yoga inculcates discipline. Apart from being therapeutic, it is an exhilarating experience harmonising the body, mind and spirit. The combination of posture, relaxation, repetitions and breathing clears the body of toxins, cleanses the mind and allows the free flow of energy. One emerges refreshed and rejuvenated after a yoga session. Yoga also helps in releasing tensions generated from repetitive mundane activities that make daily tasks unbearable. The suppleness and flexibility of the body can be regained and restored with regular practise of Yoga.

Yoga asanas are famous for being non-violent. Least amount of energy is utilised while performing the various postures. One never feels tired and exhausted at the end of a Yoga session because a lot of lubrication is created in the joints. Due to rotation, flexion or extension, the muscles have the optimum control, contraction or optimum relaxation. It is a competition between one's own body and one's own self as the practise of asanas makes one judicious in action, thought and speech.

Man grows harmoniously from the physical to the mental level and from the mental to the spiritual level. The greatest advantage of yogic postures is that it exercises the organs of our body like the lungs, glandular systems, liver, spleen, pancreas, thyroid, genitals, and urinary systems, and maintains them in perfect health all through our life span. A mere 25-30 minutes of Yoga asanas every second or third day, if not daily, is sufficient to keep a perfect, balanced health (mind and body) even during old age. One can attain a sound mind in a sound body through the practise of Yoga.

History of Yoga

Indian culture has given many gifts to the world. One of the gifts which has taken the modern world by storm is the ancient art of Yoga. The exact origins of Yoga are unknown but it is thought to be centuries old.

Yoga is referred to in the ancient texts of *Vedas* when men were interested in the quest for knowledge and self-realisation. They realised that when all the sensory organs and the mind were in complete alignment, they felt a state of calmness which they defined as yoga. Thus *tapa*, rigorous austerity, meditation and supernatural awareness became Yoga. However, this was a highly puritanical view of Yoga.

Around 200BC, Rishi Patanjali, compiled and refined the system of Yoga. He was the first person to put into writing all the verbal teachings of Yoga, which came to be known as the **Yoga Sutras**.

He laid down 8 steps of classical Yoga. They include :

* Yama   -   moral restraint
* Niyams   -   observance

* Asana   - postures
* Pranayama   - breath control
* Pratyahara - controlling the senses
* Dharna   - concentration
* Dhyana   - meditation
* Samadhi   - transconsciousness or contemplation

The first five steps which deal with the body and mind form the 'Hatha Yoga'. The latter three deal with 'Raja Yoga'. The real Yoga is a combination of Hatha and Raja. Pratyahara (fifth step) bridges the two systems together.

Asanas for Ailments

For the benefit of maintaining good health physically and mentally, one must practise all the asanas covered in detail in this book. One can derive special benefits in curing ailments by practising the asanas given in the chart below and these have to be practised only with expert guidance.

Ailments	Asanas
Acidity	Virabhadrasana, Utthita Trikonasana, Janu Sirsasana, Paschimottanasana,

	Sirsasana, Sarvang-asana.
Anaemia	Paschimottanasana, Dhanurasana, Sirs-asana, Savasana.
Appendicitis	Dhanurasana, Janu Sirsasana, Sarvang-asana, Paschimottan-asana, Sirsasana.
Arthritis (lower back)	Virabhadrasana, Utthita Trikonasana, Halasasana, Sarvang-asana.
Arthritis (Shoulder joint)	Virabhadrasana, Utthita Trikonasana, Sirsasana, Sarvang-asana.

Asthma and T.B.	ArdhaMatsyendrasana, Siddhasana, Bhujangasana, Supta Vajrasana, Janu Sirsasana, Sarvangasana, Sirsasana, Paschimottanasana.
Backache	Dhanurasana, Bhujangasana, Janu Sirsasana, Sirsasana, Sarvangasana.
Blood Pressure (High)	Padmasana, Siddh asana, Virasana, Paschimottanasana, Halasana, Janu Sirsasana.

Blood Pressure (Low)	Baddhakonasana, Padmasana, Siddhasana, Paschimottanasana, Halasana, Sirsasana.
Breathlessness	Sarvangasana, Savasana, Paschimottanasana, Halasana, Sirsasana.
Cold and Cough	Dhanurasana, Sirsasana, Sarvangasana, Paschimottanasana.
Constipation	Padahastasana, Dhanurasana, Halasana, Sirsasana, Sarvangasana, Paschimottanasana.

Diabetes	Virasana, Siddhasana, Supta Vajrasana, Ardha Matsyendrasana, Dhanurasana, Sirsasana, Janu Sirsasana, Halasana, Paschimottanasana, Savasana.
Diarrhoea	Sarvangasana, Sirsasana, Janu Sirsasana.
Epilepsy	Halasana, Sirsasana, Sarvangasana.
Headache	Paschimottanasana, Halasana, Sarvangasana, Sirsasana.
Impotency	Baddhakonasana, Padmasana, Dhanur-

	asana, Paschimott-anasana, Siddhasana, Sirsasana, Sarvang-asana, Supta Vajr-asana.
Insomnia	Sarvangasana, Sav-asana.
Kidney Problems	Vajrasana, Baddhoko-nasana, Dhanurasana, Paschimottanasana, Sarvangasana, Sirs-asana, Janu Sirsasana.
Menstrual Problems	Virasana, Baddha-konasana, Paschi-mottanasana, Supta Vajrasana, Halasana,

	Bhujangasana, Sirsasana, Sarvangasana (These asanas should not be practised during pregnancy).
Obesity	Ardha Matsyendrasana, Supta Vajrasana, Dhanurasana, Paschimottanasana.
Paralysis	Tadasana, Virabhadrasana, Padmasana, Virasana Siddhasana, Utthita Trikonasana, Sirsasana, Halasana, Savasana (These

	asanas should be done with the help of expert guidance only).
Rheumatism in joints	Paschimottanasana, Sirsasana, Sarvangasana.
Spinal Displacements	Tadasana, Virabhadrasana, Dhanurasana, Paschimottanasana, Utthita Trikonasana, Supta Vajrasana.

Sitting Asanas

We often tend to sit lazily on our bottom, caving in the lower spine and dropping the chest forward. This gives an ugly hunch and due to bad posture the lower back often aches. The asanas under the sitting category lead to several advantages.

* It inculcates the discipline to sit erect.
* The regular practise of these asanas make the joints and muscles of the legs supple.
* These asanas help in preventing sprains or pulls caused due to lack

of adequate movements or exercise.

* The asanas are particularly helpful to those engaged in standing for long hours and those suffering from backaches.

Those having difficulty in sitting without support may practise the asanas by aligning the bottom to a wall. This helps to keep the back upright.

Padmasana

This asana resembles a Lotus.

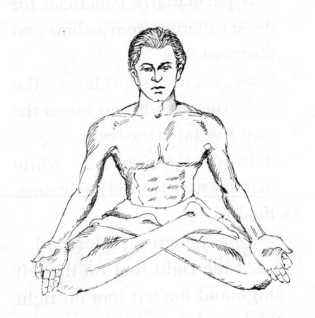

* The Padmasana is useful for everyone.
* It is particularly beneficial for those suffering from asthma and insomnia.
* This asana stimulates the endocrine glands and burns the excessive fat in the body.
* It is ideally practised while chanting mantras and meditating.

Method
* Sit with legs stretched forward.
* Keep the right foot on the left thigh and the left foot on right thigh.
* Rest the left hand on the left knee, the right hand on the right knee,

and join the thumb with the index finger of both hands respectively.

* Retain the head and back in an erect posture, and look straight.
* Remain in this state for 20 seconds, breathing normally.
* Repeat.

Time Required: 30 seconds

Repetition : Once

Sum up: Initially you may find difficulty in keeping the feet on the thighs but with practice and repetition you can achie e the Padmasana pose easily.

Siddhasana

This asana is performed by the *Siddhas* (semi-divine beings). This asana awakens the Kundalini Shakti, and purifies the tubular channels.

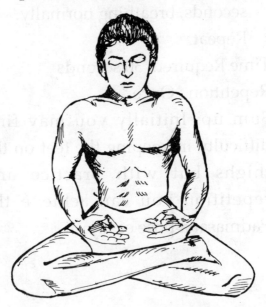

* This asana helps to cure indigestion, heart ailments, asthma and diabetes.
* The mind also becomes attentive and alert.

Method

* Sit with legs stretched forward.
* Bend the left leg, and place it near the perineum. The sole of the left foot is placed under the right thigh.
* Bend the right leg, place the right foot over the left ankle, and the heel of the right foot at the root of the genitals.
* Maintain the spine, neck and head in a straight, upright posture.

* Place both hands near the thigh joints, slightly bent at elbows on either side; join the middle fingers and thumbs respectively.
* Slowly bend the neck, look downwards and allow the chin to touch the bottom of the throat.
* Breathe normally, remain in this pose for 30 seconds.
* Repeat.

Time Required: 40 seconds

Repetition : Once

Sum up: As this asana cures the stiffness of the joints of the loin, one may feel some pain initially. Condition improves with practice and repetition.

Dandasana

Danda means stick and this is a basic sitting asana.

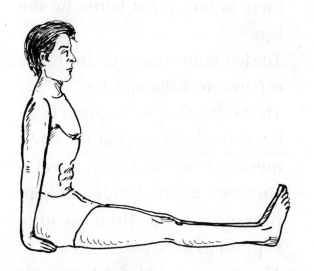

* This asana is a great relief to people suffering from arthritis, and rheumatism.

* As the legs are extended forward there is no weight borne by the legs.

* The joints are more free due to the expansion of the muscles.

* The body gets good support from the extended legs, and the chest muscles near the armpit are also stretched as the hands are kept pressed on the floor to give support to the chest.

* This asana is helpful to people suffering from asthmatic attacks and breathlessness.

Method

* Sit with legs stretched forward.
* Place the palms beside the body on the floor.
* The buttocks, bottom of the thighs, calf muscles and heels are kept in a straight line on the floor and the back, shoulder, neck and head are kept upright.
* Stretch the legs forward keeping them pressed on the floor, and flex the knuckles of the toes.
* Do not allow the back to bend. Pull in the abdomen slightly, and expand the chest.
* Remain in this pose for 30 seconds.

*   Repeat.

Time required: 35 seconds

Repetition: Once

Sum up: The legs do not bear any weight as one is sitting and stretching the legs and thus helping the knee and ankle muscles to stretch and expand. People suffering from asthma or spinal ailments may be able to do this asana by giving support to the torso against the wall.

Baddhakonasana

This is a cobbler pose.

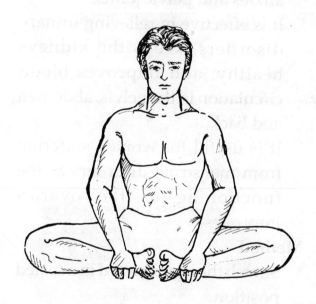

* This asana gives firmness to the thighs and stretches the knees, ankles and pelvic joints.
* It is effective in relieving urinary disorders, keeps the kidneys healthy, and improves blood circulation in the pelvis, abdomen and back.
* It is useful for women suffering from menstrual disorders as the functioning of the ovaries improves.

Method
* Stretch the legs forward in a seated position.
* Fold the legs at the knee and bring the feet together, and clasp the feet with the palms.

34

* Slowly rest the knees down on the floor till a tight stretch is felt at the thighs and joints.
* Remain in this pose for 30 seconds.
* Breathe normally.
* Repeat.

Time required: 40 seconds.

Repetition : Once

Sum up: This asana is a boon to women, particularly pregnant women. They will experience less pain at the time of labour and also be free from varicose veins. It may be difficult to make the knees touch the floor but continuous repetition would enable easy achievement of the posture.

Virasana

This asana means warrior pose and the practice of this makes one brave and adventurous.

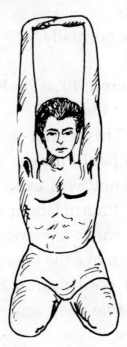

* This asana brings relief to people having arthritis and rheumatism by reducing pain and stiffness in the knees and ankles.
* Those feeling heavy after eating may do the asana immediately to feel lighter.
* It helps in enhancing the movement of the chest for better respiration and hence is ideal for singers.

Method
* Sit on the buttocks with the knees folded and kept together.
* Fold the legs at the knees with the toes pointing backwards, and rest the knees and toes on the floor.

* Allow the palms to rest on the knees.
* Bend the chest a little forward so that the weight of the body is on the knee.
* Stretch the abdomen upright, keeping the back erect.
* Breathe normally.
* Extend the hands in front of the chest, interlock the fingers and open out the palms.
* Raise the hand above the head, keeping the upper arm behind the ears and palms facing the sky.
* Remain in this posture for 30 seconds, breathing normally.
* Repeat.

Time required: 45 seconds

Repetition : Once

Sum up: This asana can be performed even after meals in order to relieve the heavy feeling. Initially this asana can be practised by placing folded blankets under the buttocks or resting the buttocks on the feet, to give a cushioning effect to the buttocks.

Sukhasana

This asana improves body posture.
It is the easiest asana for a beginner.

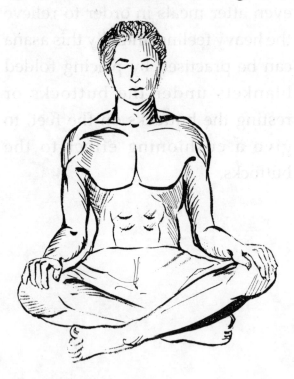

* It improves blood circulation.
* It calms the mind and helps in meditation.
* It is important to remain quiet during this asana.

Method

* Cross the legs at the ankles.
* Place the heels below the thighs.
* Place the palms on the knees.
* Relax the elbows.
* The neck, head and the spine should be maintained straight.
* Breathe normally.
* Eyes should be closed and one should concentrate on breathing.

Time required : 7-10 minutes.

Sum up: If you face difficulty in keeping the spine erect, you could take the support of the wall.

Gomukhasana

"Gomukh" means cow-head.

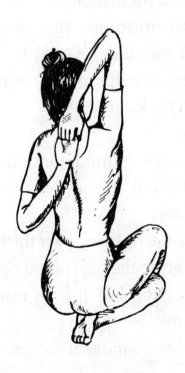

* This asana improves blood circulation, particularly in and around the armpits.
* It strengthens the muscles, tendons and ligaments of the knees. It helps people suffering from backaches.

Method
* Sit on the ground, place the heel of the left leg under the right buttock.
* Place the right leg over the left leg and bring the heel of the right leg under the left hip as much as possible.
* Place the hands on the knees.

44

* The body and the spine should be kept straight.
* Close the eyes and concentrate on breathing.
* To achieve complete Gomukhasana place the right arm over the shoulder, so that the elbow is at the same level as the head.
* Place the left arm behind the back.
* Try and hold the fingers of both hands.
* Breathe normally and repeat.

Ustrasana

This is the camel pose.

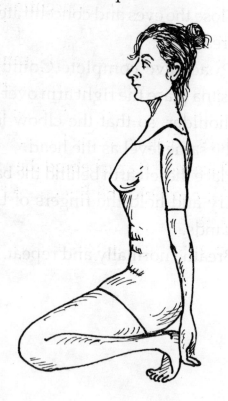

* This asana is meant for women.
* This asana stretches and expands the spine and promotes blood circulation.
* It exercises the muscles of the torso, thighs and neck.
* It improves the functioning of the ovaries, thyroid and other endocrine glands.

Method
* Sit on the ground in the kneeling position. The body should be supported on the toes and the knees.
* Bend backwards.
* Hold the heels with the hands. The fingers of the hand should

point outwards and the thumbs should point towards the toes.
* While inhaling, gradually lift the pelvis. Press the upper torso, both outwards and upwards and bend the neck downwards. The arms should be kept straight.
* While exhaling return to the kneeling position.

Time Required: 60 seconds

Repetition: Five times

Vakrasana

This asana helps in reducing obesity.

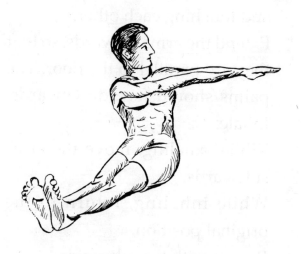

* It corrects minor displacements of the vertebrae.
* It also gently twists the spine.

Method

* Sit with legs extended forward and touching each other.
* Extend the arms forwards, so that they are parallel to the floor. The palms should face downwards. Inhale.
* While exhaling, move the arms sidewards.
* While inhaling, return to the original position.
* Repeat with the other side.

Time required: 90 seconds

Repetition: Five times (alternately)

Standing Asanas

It is important to stand erect by distributing our body weight evenly on both legs. These asanas inculcate in us the basic activity familiar to all. Standing helps in the following ways :

* Strengthens and softens the muscles, bones and joints, by removing rigidity in the joints of the legs.
* The extra fat around the waist, hips, thighs is burned.
* It provides relief to people suffering from asthma, arthritis

rheumatic pain, spondylitis and pains arising from doing sedentary work.

Tadasana

This asana teaches us the correct posture. Everyone can do this asana.

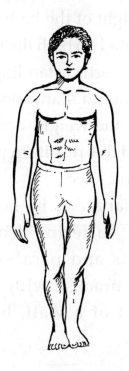

* From heels to the head, the body is maintained in a horizontally aligned position.
* The weight of the body is evenly distributed on both the feet. Often due to incorrect standing posture, one tends to stand on one side putting the weight only on that side and this results in pain of the ankle and knee.
* This asana can be helpful for people suffering from heart ailments and paralysis. They should practise with adequate support of a wall, handle or window.

Method

* Bring the feet together. Heels, big toes and knees should touch each other.
* Keep the hands straight beside the body.
* The back, shoulder, neck, chest and abdomen should be kept straight and erect.
* Look straight. Breathe normally.
* Remain in the same posture for 30 seconds.
* Repeat.

Time required: 30 seconds.

Repetition: Once

Sum up : Everyone needs to walk, so this asana is very important, and cannot be omitted. Regular practice enables one to have the right standing pose, eliminating drooping shoulders, sagging abdomen or caved back.

Vrukshasana

Vruksha means tree and in this asana the body gives the appearance of the shape of a tree.

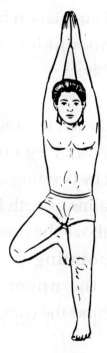

*   While toning all the joints, this asana maintains flexibility of the arms and limbs and develops a shapely chest.
*   The blood circulation in the toes, knees and ankles improves considerably.

Method

*   Stand on the left leg and place the heel of the right leg on the inner thigh joint by bending at the knee.
*   Join the palms of both hands and lift them above the head with the fingers pointing at the sky, ensuring the upper arms are placed behind the ears.

* Elongate and straighten the elbows.
* Breathe normally.
* Remain in the same posture for 20 seconds.
* Repeat the same procedure on the right side.
* Repeat all over once.

Time required: 50 seconds

Repetition: Once

Sum up : This asana can also be done by taking the support of a wall.

Utthita Trikonasana

Utthita means stretched, *trikona* means triangle.

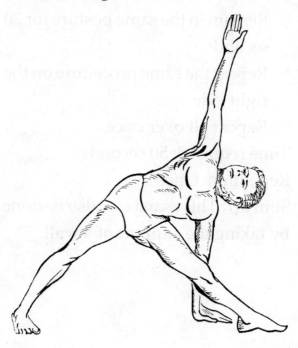

* A perfect coordination of the hand and leg is achieved in this asana.
* Minor defects in the limbs are corrected and ligaments become flexible.
* The organs in the pelvic region are benefited and people find relief from gastritis and acidity. Women find relief from menstrual disorders.

Method

* Stand with feet apart.
* Keep the left sole firmly planted on the floor and turn the right foot sideways.

* Extend your palms on either side of the body, stretching the arms parallel to the floor.
* Breathe normally.
* Slowly exhale and bend on the right side and allow the palm to touch the floor behind the right heel.
* A slight push of the right buttock forward would make the bending easier.
* Slightly move the head upwards and look at the tip of the fingers extended up towards the sky.
* Ensure to keep the weight of the body on the left heel and the right knee.

* Breathe normally.
* Remain in this pose for 30 seconds.
* While raising the body upwards, inhale.
* Repeat the whole posture on the left side.

Time required : 1 minute 20 seconds.

Repetition: Once

Sum up : This asana calls for correct coordinated stretch movements of various parts of the body viz. legs, hands, back, abdomen, head, pelvic organs. Be very careful while performing this asana.

Virabhadrasana

This asana means warrior pose.

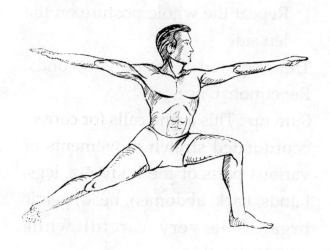

* The hip joints, knees, groins become flexible and relaxed.
* The rigid shoulder and neck joints get flexible and supple.
* People suffering from defective spinal column find relief.
* The accumulated fat around the hips gets burned. The misplaced uterus also gets corrected.

Method

* Stand with the feet apart.
* Extend the arms on the sides parallel to the floor with palms facing the floor.
* Slowly lift the forefoot of the right leg, turn the leg sideways towards

the right side, right knee facing the right side and then place the foot on the floor.

* Bend the right knee in such a way that the outer knee and the heel of that leg are in the same line and form a perpendicular line to the floor.

* Turn the head towards the right and look towards the right side. Remain in this posture for 30 seconds.

* Breathe normally.

* Repeat the whole exercise on the left side also.

Time required: 1 minute 20 seconds.

Repetition: Once

Sum up: The asana helps in developing endurance capacity. While back muscles get strengthened, the abdominal and chest muscles also get toned.

Padahastasana

This asana helps in reducing the superfluous fat of the body.

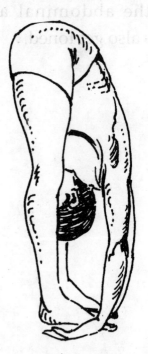

* Spinal, abdominal and calf muscles get toned. The body gets a good shape.
* This asana improves digestion.
* Organs like the liver, kidneys, and stomach function better.

Method
* Stand straight keeping the hands on either side.
* Keep some gap between the feet; keep the heels and knees together.
* Extend the arms in front at the shoulder level.
* Slowly exhale and bend forward without bending the knees and allow the palms to hold the respective ankles.

* Breathe normally.
* Remain in this pose for 10 seconds.
* Repeat.

Time required: 20 seconds.

Repetition: Once

Sum up : The superfluous fat in the body gets burned. Since this asana works on the arms and limbs, any unevenness in the length of the leg due to fracture in the leg can be corrected.

Chakrasana

Chakra means wheel.

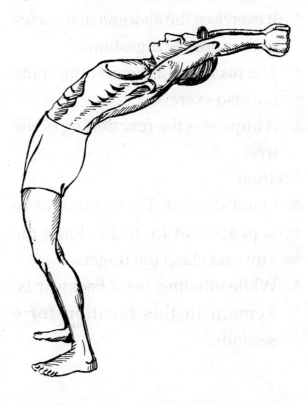

* This asana exercises the back muscles.
* It exercises the abdominal muscles and improves digestion.
* The neck, shoulder and the spine are also exercised.
* It improves the functioning of the liver.

Method
* Stand straight. The feet should be kept apart at 18" to 20". Raise the arm and clasp the fingers.
* While inhaling, bend backwards.
* Remain in this position for 6 seconds.

* While exhaling bend forward. The knees should not be bent.
* Gradually try to touch the ground and bring the head closer to the knees.
* Slowly inhale and straighten the torso. Pause.

Repetition: Five times.

Time required: 50 seconds

Forward Bending Asanas

As the name suggests, these asanas have forward body movements. The muscles of the back are extended forward.

The asanas help in the following ways:

* The back gets stretched and gains strength, flexibility and suppleness.

* It also improves the functioning of the abdominal organs, thereby improving digestion.

*   These asanas are effective in maintaining a normal flow during menstruation.
*   Back pain is considerably reduced if these asanas are regularly performed.

Paschimottanasana

Paschima means west, *ut* means intensity and *tana* means stretch.

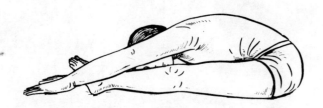

* Being foremost of all the forward bending asanas, in this asana the entire back muscle is made to stretch forward. There is a flow of *prana* through the important organs of the body.

* It activates the liver, kidneys, bladder and pancreas and hence the digestive, excretory, and glandular organs function properly. The brain also rests.

* The asana also makes the reproductive organs healthier, reducing the chance of impotency.

Method

* Sit down with both legs extended forwards.

* Keep the heels, back of the legs and buttocks firmly rested on the floor.
* Extend the palms to take a firm grip of the soles, keep the upper spine slightly bent without curving the back or drooping the chest; pull the abdomen upwards.
* Slightly bend the elbows and exhale; slowly lower the torso and head.
* Rest the forehead on the legs. The tip of the nose should touch the knees, the back is to be kept straight, and the elbows should touch the floor besides the shin of the legs on either side.

78

* If the lower side of the legs are pressed downwards and the upper part of the legs are pulled upwards, then a better posture casn be attained.
* Remain in this pose for 30 seconds.
* While raising the head upwards, inhale.
* Repeat.

Time required: 50 seconds.

Repetition: Once

Sum up: In case of difficulty in reaching and then resting the head on the leg, some folded blankets may be kept on the legs but never attempt to lower the torso by curving your back and drooping the chest.

Janu Sirsasana

Janu means knee and *sirsa* means the head.

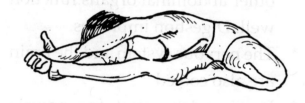

* In this asana the Kundalini gets awakened and body and mind become alert and stronger.
* The digestive organs are exercised and toned.
* Liver, spleen, kidneys and all other abdominal organs function well. Digestion improves.
* The nervous system and the brain are also cooled.
* It provides relief for people suffering from headache, migraine, high blood pressure, and diabetes.

Method
* Sit with legs extended forwards.

* Bend the left leg at the knee, place the heel near the perineum allowing the left toe to touch the inner side of the right thigh.

* The right leg is stretched and extended forwards. The left knee is extended outward in line with the thigh joint so that, the two legs make a fine obtuse angle.

* Hold the sole of the extended leg with the palms while keeping the lower side of the leg firmly on the floor.

* Bend the torso forward enabling the head to touch the extended leg without curving the back or the chest, and exhale.

* Remain for 30 seconds in this pose.
* Repeat with the other leg.

Time required: 1 minute 30 seconds

Repetition: Once

Sum up: It is easier to practise this asana when the bowels are empty.

Triangmukhaikapada
Paschimottanasana

Triang means three parts of the leg, viz, feet, knees and buttocks and these are used in this forward stretch asana.

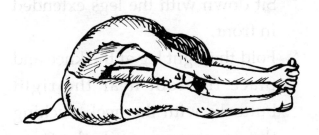

* In this asana, the knees become highly supple and flexible and the ligaments are also extended.
* The abdominal organs are exercised as the back is made to bend and stretch.

Method
* Sit down with the legs extended in front.
* Fold the right leg at the knee and place the foot near the right buttocks with the heel touching the perenium and the toes pointing backwards. Slightly tilt the right buttock but do not shift the weight of the body to the left

buttock. Ensure that both the
buttocks are resting on the floor.

* Extend the hands and clasp the left
  sole with both the palms.

* Without curving the back or chest
  bring the torso down by slightly
  curving the elbows, and exhale
  when you come down.

* Place the forehead on the knee and
  keep the left lower leg pressed on
  the floor. Do not bend the left
  knee, keep it straight. Remain in
  this posture for 45 seconds,
  breathing normally.

* Repeat the same with the other leg
  and complete the exercise.

Time required : 2 minutes
Repetition : Once
Sum up : Care must be taken while doing the asana, as incorrect posture may damage the knee ligaments or back muscles.

Pranatasana

This asana is the child's pose.

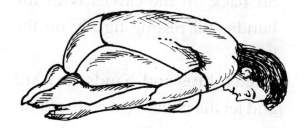

* It relaxes the body between asanas or asana sequences.

Method

* Kneel on the floor.
* Keep the hands in front of the knees, resting lightly on the knees.
* Sit back on the calves with the hands still resting lightly on the knees.
* Stretch hips and hands forward and let the palms rest on the floor. Keep the shoulders relaxed.
* Let the head touch the floor.
* Relax in this position for 10 seconds, breathing normally.

Time Required: 30 seconds
Repetition: Once
Sum up : This asana relaxes the body and calms the mind. It is a sort of break between the asana sequences.

Backward Bending Asanas

These asanas have backward body movements. The muscles of the back are bent backwards. These asanas help in the following ways:

* They help to cure backaches and spinal disorders.
* When the back is bent backwards the abdomen is fully exercised, nourished and blood circulation improves.
* These asanas strengthen the ovaries and uterus thereby curing any menstrual disorder.

Bhujangasana

Bhujanga means a serpent. This asana resembles a cobra reared up on its caudal support with the hood fully expanded.

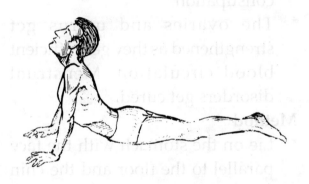

* With this asana back pain and spinal disorders are cured.
* Pressure is exerted on the internal organs of the abdomen, and the excreta is pushed to the anus, and helps people suffering from constipation.
* The ovaries and uterus get strengthened as they get sufficient blood circulation. Menstrual disorders get cured.

Method
* Lie on the stomach with the face parallel to the floor and the chin touching the chest.
* Keep all the muscles relaxed and place the palms of both the hands on the floor below the shoulders.

*   Inhaling, lift the head and torso upwards by pressing the palms downwards on the floor. Keep the legs pressed on the floor and stretch the legs, soles facing the sky and toes touching the floor.
*   The shoulder and back muscles get completely stretched and the abdomen gets elongated.
*   Hold your breath.
*   Remain in this posture for 20 seconds.
*   Exhale.
*   Come down.
*   Repeat.

Time required: 40 seconds
Repetition: Once
Sum up: This is a beneficial asana for people suffering from back pain. The neck and chest muscles are exercised and the shape of the body improves.

Dhanurasana

Dhanush means a bow. In this asana the hands are used like a bow string to pull the head, trunk and legs up and the final pose resembles a bent bow.

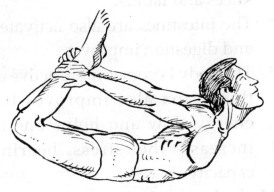

* As the back is bent backwards, the abdomen gets elongated and is fully exercised and nourished, and receives proper blood circulation.
* This asana also cures a spinal hump and rheumatism of the legs, knees and hands.
* The intestines are also activated and digestion improves.
* The body becomes more active as this asana also improves the energy flow and helps one to increase the stress bearing capacity.

Method

* Lie on your stomach. With your face parallel to the floor and your muscles relaxed.

* Place the arms beside the body on the floor.
* Slightly bend your knees and lift your legs upwards and extend your hands and clasp the ankles.
* Exhale and lift your head and chest away from the floor.
* Tighten the hand on the leg and inhale. Keep the lower abdomen and pelvic region firmly on the floor, and knees joined.
* Hold your breath and remain like this for 20 seconds.

Time required: 30 seconds

Repetition: Once

Sum up: It is important to do this asana on an empty stomach as the whole body is resting on the stomach. For a better pose slightly rock the body from left to right and forward and backwards in the final posture.

Twisting Asanas

The asanas in this category teach the art of the lateral twisting of the spine. The back is made to twist along with the vertical extension and this gives relief from backaches. There is stimulation of the abdominal organs and better digestion, absorption and assimilation.

Ardha Matsyendrasana

Ardha means half and Matsyendranath was the first yogi to teach this asana to the world.

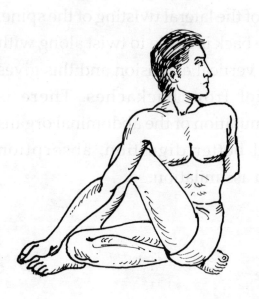

* This asana stimulates the appetite and awakens the Kundalini.
* It also increases the elasticity of the back muscles and abdominal muscles and improves blood circulation too.

Method

* Sit on the floor, bend the right leg at the knee and place the right heel near the buttock below the perenium.
* Bend the left knee, place the left ankle on the outer side of the right knee.
* Rest the right armpit on the outer side of the left thigh.

* Gently push the knee backwards to touch the back of the armpit and hold the toe of the left foot with the right hand.
* Exhaling, twist the torso backwards to the farthest possible, putting force on the left shoulder.
* Turn the head also towards the left and look ahead. The neck and left shoulder should be aligned.
* Move left hand backwards and hold the right thigh.
* Keep the back, abdomen and chest erect.
* Remain in this posture for 30 seconds.

*   Breathe normally.

*   Repeat the steps on the other side.

Time required: 1 minute 40 seconds

Repetition: Once

Sum up : Be careful while twisting the back. Women suffering from leucorrhea, menorrhagia, and metrohagia should restrain from doing this exercise. However, this asana tones up the kidneys, intestines, pancreas, liver and spleen.

Garudasana

This is the eagle pose.

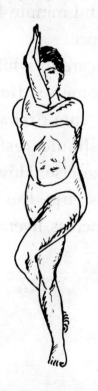

* This asana helps to loosen the joints by stretching the muscles of the shoulders, elbows, wrists, hips, knees and ankles.

Method

* Stand erect. Lift the right leg and twist it around the other, both near the hip-joint and the knee.

* Lock the ankle of the left leg with the toe of the twisted right leg. This is done to avoid possible release.

* Exhale and balance on the left leg. Gradually, increase the pressure on the toehold till the maximum twist is obtained.

* Twine the arms together to obtain a twist.
* The wrists should also be twined together with the palms facing each other.
* Inhale and return to the original position.

Time required: 20 seconds

Repetition: 3 times on each side, alternately

Sum up: Regular practice increases the flexibility and suppleness of the limbs.

Lying Asanas

These asanas are performed lying down. The asanas give relief from fatigue, stress and work pressure. It soothes the body and rests the wandering brain.

* These asanas are particularly helpful to people suffering from insomnia due to stomach upsets, indigestion, heavy and bloated feeling in the abdomen or mental tension, breathlessness, fatigue, nervousness, depression.

 * However, people suffering from psychological disturbances and

arthritis must perform these only by keeping a back-rest.

* These asanas should be performed only at the last. They should never be performed between other asanas as there would be a loss of harmony in the nervous system.

Savasana

In this asana, all the layers from the skin to the innermost core are calmed.

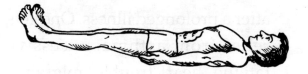

* In this asana, all the parts of the body, the organs, muscles, bones and nerves, brain, mind get relaxed totally.
* As there is absolute concentration on the breathing and its rhythmic flow, one feels soothed and refreshed, and can recoup faster after a prolonged illness. One gets relief from asthma, excessive fatigue, heart trouble, migraine, insomnias and nervous weakness.
* Those suffering from backache may do the asana on a chair.

Method
* Lie straight on the back.

* Keep the hands on either side of the body, a little away from the thigh, palms facing the sky.
* Part the legs, leaving a gap between them.
* Let the heels touch each other and toes be far apart.
* Lightly clasp the fists and close the eyes.
* Breathe slowly.
* Concentrate on the ankles and relax them.
* Concentrate on the calves and relax them. Concentrate on the thighs and hips and relax them.
* Gradually concentrate on the waist, back, abdomen, chest and relax.

* Relax the fingers, lower arms, upper arms and shoulders. The neck muscles and facial muscles should also be completely relaxed. Concentrate and relax the head.
* Inhale and exhale slowly and rhythmically, taking deep breathes, and exhaling fully.
* When exhaling, relax the brain by concentrating on the breathing.
* Remain in this state for one minute.
* Slowly open your eyes and emerge thoroughly relaxed.

Supta Vajrasana

Supta means lying down.

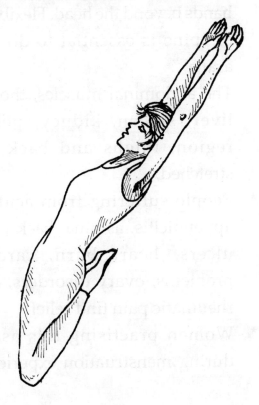

* In this asana you will be reclining back on the floor, extending the hands beyond the head. Flexibility of spine is essential to do this asana.
* The abdominal muscles, thorax, liver, spleen, kidney, pelvic region, thighs and back are stretched.
* People suffering from acidity, appendicitis, asthma, back pain, ulcers, heart burn, cardiac problems, ovary disorders, and rheumatic pain find relief.
* Women practising this asana during menstruation experience

comfort. This asana activates the pancreatic cells, increasing the blood supply to the pancreas, making it function normally. Hence it is very useful for diabetics.

* There is a stimulation of all the glands resulting in a feeling of health.

* This asana also gives relief from indigestion, gastritis, constipation and piles.

Method

* In the first part one has to attain the Vajrasana. Sit down with legs extended forward.

* Fold the legs at the knee and place the heels besides the buttocks on either side.
* Give support to the body at the knees and ankles.
* Breathe normally.
* Place the palms by the side of the feet, exhaling, and supporting the elbow, lower the torso and rest on the elbows.
* Lower the head first allowing the upper head to rest on the floor.
* Stretch further by resting the back of the head.
* Ensure that the knees, shin, thighs, buttocks, shoulders and back of the head are firmly resting on the floor.

* Stretch the arms over the head, behind the ears, and keep the palms facing the sky.
* Breathe normally.
* Remain in this pose for 30 seconds. Repeat.

Time required: 50 seconds.

Repetition: Once

Sum up : This asana can be helpful to athletes and all those who have to stand or walk for long hours. People suffering from arthritis and slipped disc may do the asana with the aid of a backrest.

Yastik Asana
This means a stick pose.

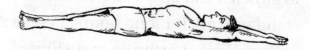

* This asana stretches the entire body.
* It helps to increase height.
* It also helps to cure backache.

Method
* Lie on the back on the ground. Place the arms over the head. The arms should touch the floor and be placed in a relaxed manner.
* Inhale. While inhaling stretch the arms, legs, hands, and feet in the opposite direction as much as possible.
* Remain in this position for 6 seconds. Exhale and come back to normal position.

Repetition : 4 times

Time required: 20 seconds

Shalabhasana

This is a locust pose. This asana has two variations.

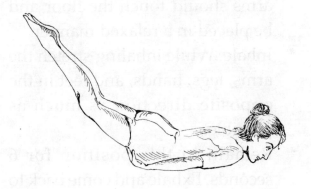

* This asana strengthens the muscles of the legs and the lower back.
* It also benefits people suffering from rheumatic pains in the lower back and hips.
* It reduces the excess weight around the hips, waist and abdomen.
* It cures menstrual disorders.

Method

Variation I

* Lie on the stomach. The chin should touch the floor.
* Extend the arms along the sides. Clench the fists and inhale. The hands could also be placed under the thighs.

* While exhaling, raise the right leg as much as you can, and slightly press the clenched fists.
* The head should not be raised from the ground and the knees should not be bent.
* While inhaling lower the leg and relax.

Time required: 30 seconds

Repetition: 4 times

Variation II

* Place the palms underneath the thighs. Inhale.
* While exhaling raise both the legs.
* While inhaling lower the legs and relax.

Repetition : Each variation should be
                done four times.
Time required: 30 seconds

Pavanmuktasana

This asana helps people suffering from constipation and flatulence.

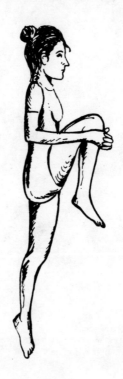

* This asana has two variations.
* This asana exercises the various joints like the hip, knee and ankle joints.

Method

Variation I

* Lie on the ground with the arms on the sides and inhale.
* Raise one leg and while exhaling fold the leg at the knee joint and hold the knee with the hands.
* Press the knee on the stomach and keep the other leg straight.
* Remain in this posture for four seconds.
* While inhaling return to the original position.

127

*   Repeat with the other leg.

Time required: 20 seconds

Repetition: Once

Varitation II

*   Fold both the legs at the knee joints. The arms should be folded around the legs.

*   Remain in this posture till the suspension of breath.

*   The knees and feet should remain together.

*   While inhaling release both the legs. One must rest before repeating the exercise.

Time required: 30 seconds

Repetition: Once

Head Postures

In this asana one is head over heels (upside down) and with regular practise one can easily master this art. To master this art one has to attain perfection in balancing the body. One should be able to do the standing asanas correctly and precisely by achieving absolute muscle control. By developing the skill to keep the body balance, without any growing tension to the muscles, one starts to feel lighter.

* These asanas provide relief from stress and tiredness.

* The supply of blood to the brain improves, thereby improving memory power and intelligence.
* The most important advantage of this asana is that it calms the mind.

Sirsasana

Sirsa means head and this head stand
asana is known as the king of asanas.

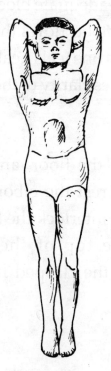

* This asana enables the two important glands responsible for growth viz. pineal and pituitary to receive adequate blood supply.
* As pure blood flows through the brain cells one feels healthier, and experiences clarity of thought and vigour.

Method

* Kneel on the floor, and leaning forward, rest the elbows on the floor and interlock the fingers.
* Keep the top of the head in between the clasped hands and elbows.

* Exhale, and slowly lift the legs first resting on the toes and then stretching upwards, toes pointing towards the sky.
* Remain in the head stand posture for 20 seconds.
* Breathe normally.

Time required: 30 seconds

Repetition: Once

Sum up: This asana may be performed slowly increasing the duration of keeping the legs in the raised position. It must be done on an empty stomach. However, a cup of milk or light snack may be consumed after completion of the asana.

Sarvangasana

The meaning of this asana is 'all parts pose' as all the parts of the body are thoroughly exercised.

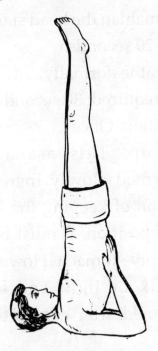

* There is a perfect union of the mind, the body and the soul.
* The firm lock of the chin helps in pure blood supply to the thyroid and para-thyroid glands.
* The body is in an inverted posture, and so it feels light, and the brain sublime.
* People suffering from asthma, bronchitis and throat problems get tremendous relief; bowel movements are easy too.
* This asana works well even for those suffering from urinary disorders, displaced uterus, menstrual trouble, hernia and piles.

* The haemoglobin level in the blood also improves. In other words, this is an ideal strength-giving exercise, and expands the span of youth when practised regularly.

Method

* Lie on the floor on the back with the body fully stretched.
* Fill your lungs with air; inhale deeply. Lift the legs from the thigh to the toe upwards.
* Raise the hips and trunk along with the legs in a slow continuous movement, supporting the back with both the hands. Only the

back of the head and shoulders are kept on the floor firmly and the entire weight of the body rests on them.

* Keep the legs in an upright pose, toes pointing upwards to the sky, and look towards the toes. Place the chin at the bottom of the neck.

* Remain for 30 seconds in this pose.

* Breathe normally.

Time required: 45 seconds

Repetition: Once

Sum up : People suffering from high blood pressure should not attempt this asana. Beginners may do this

asana by taking somebody's help to
hold the leg upright till they can do
it on their own .

Halasana

Hala means plough.

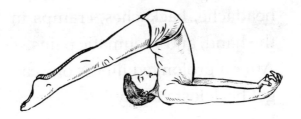

* The blood vessels of the back muscles, spine and nerves get nourished, and it instantly relaxes the eyes and brain by removing the tension in those areas.

* People get relief from migraine headache, backaches, cramps in the hand, and rheumatic pains.

* After a prolonged illness one can get back lost vitality.

* Women must avoid this asana during menstruation and advanced pregnancy.

Method

* Lie on the floor on the back.

* Place the hands stretched beside the body, palms facing the floor.

* Keep the legs together and stretch.
* Inhale.
* Raise both legs together, keeping the inner side of the legs touching each other, and do not bend the knees or back.
* Lower the legs behind the head to touch the floor. The toes should point outwards.
* Keep the chin at the base of the neck.
* Breathe normally.
* Remain in this pose for 20 seconds.

Time required: 45 seconds

Repetition: Once

Sum up: This asana instantly relieves fatigue. It also gets rid of heaviness and gives energy to the body enabling one to perform better.

Kriyas

Personal hygiene

The ancient yogis felt that physical activity was not sufficient to maintain a healthy body and mind. Proper care of the body and its various organs was necessary for maintaining good health.

* Hatha Yoga is a type of yoga that cleanses the internal system. It is a method of hygiene or *shuddhi*. It is also called ghatsya yoga or physiological yoga.

* The cleansing is a six-fold process. It cleans both internal and external organs like the ears, nose, eyes, the sinuses, the food pipe, and the intestines.

* These Kriyas help the body to get rid of pathogenic metabolites. The Kriyas keep the body free from disease.

Tratak

This asana exercises the eye muscles. It cures minor eye defects and improves concentration.

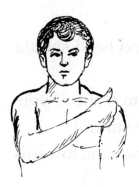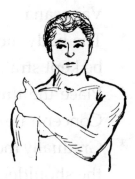

There are two methods of doing this asana:

(a) The left shoulder gaze.

(b) The right shoulder gaze.

Method

* Sit in the position of Sukhasana or Vajrasana.

* The body, neck and head should be kept straight.

* Place the thumb in front of you. Concentrate on the thumb.

* Gradually move the hand towards the shoulder.

* The eyes should be kept wide open, and should be fixed on the thumb nail. The head should not be turned.

* Repeat the exercise for the other shoulder.
* Close the eyes each time to rest them.

Repetition: 3 times alternately.

Nasal Gaze

It improves concentration and exercises the eye muscles.

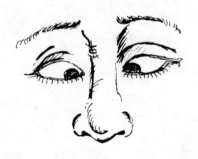

Method

* Sit on the ground.
* Fix the eyes on the tip of the nose. The tyes should be kept wide open.
* Shift the gaze of the eyes to a point between the eyebrows.
* Whenever the eyes are tired, cover them with the palms.
* Repetition: 3 times with each gaze.

Diet and Yoga

Diet is considered very important in yoga. It is believed that diet not only affects the physical condition but also the mental condition.

Diet can be of three kinds:

Rajasi, tamasi and *sattvic.*

Rajasi means kingly. It comprises non-vegetarian dishes. It is a high-protein and high-energy yielding diet.

* This diet is not recommended by yoga practitioners as it leads to an increase in body weight.

* It creates a feeling of heaviness, lethargy and a general lack of interest.

* This diet also arouses passion.

The *Tamasi* diet comprises both vegetarian and non-vegetarian dishes.

* This diet consists of a lot of spices like chilli and pepper, stale food, and cold, reheated food.
* This diet is also not recommended by yoga practitioners. It is believed that it makes a person quarrelsome and intolerant.

Sattvic diet is pure vegetarian with very little spices. This diet is recommended by yoga practitioners as it is:

* Well-balanced.
* It is easy to digest.

* The cholesterol level in the *sattvic* diet is low.
* Green and leafy vegetables which are a part of this diet help to maintain the hormonal balance in the body.

Selection of food stuffs according to yogic diet.

Food Groups	Food stuff
Cereal	Wheat, rice, jowar, bajra. They are a good source of carbohydrates.
Milk	Milk in itself is a complete meal. Milk

products such as butter, buttermilk, curd, cheese are full of protein, minerals and vitamins

Pulses   Pulses are a source of protein. Soyabean is a good source of protein. It also contains a good amount of iron and vitamins.

Vegetables   Among all the vegetables, yogis recommend certain vegetables which are a good source of vitamins and minerals.

Spinach	Spinach is a good source of iron, vitamins, calcium, and amino-acids. Lettuce, radish, and fenu-greek also contain minerals and vita-mins.
Ladies Fingers	This vegetable is very useful for genito-urinary organs, and in stomach disorders.
Wild Snake gourd	This is good for energy and strength.
Brinjal	This vegetable helps people suffering from liver ailments.

Bittergourd	This helps to purify the blood. It is recommended for people suffering from rheumatism and diseases of the spleen and liver.
Roots and Tubers	Potatoes, beetroot, and carrots are good sources of carbohydrates.
Sugar and jaggery	Jaggery is a good source of carbohydrate and energy.
Fruits	All kinds of fruits are recommended as they are a good source of vitamins.

Dry fruit	Yoga practitioners also recommend dry fruits, like, dates, figs, raisins, and almonds as they are a good source of vitamin.
Oil and Fats	Mustard, sesame, and sunflower oil should be used for cooking as they contain unsatu-rated fats.
Spices and alochol	These are considered harmful for the body.
Tea and coffee	Tea and coffee are not considered good for the body. They should be avoided after meals.

The body needs of each individual differs. What is suitable for one may not be suitable for the other. Therefore one should work out a diet that fulfils one's body needs.

An ideal diet should be :

* Energy giving.

* Health-promoting.

* Balanced – it should consist of grains, milk, cereals, yoghurt, cottage cheese, green leafy vegetables, salads, fresh fruits, etc.

Yogis recommend that one should eat only what is necessary to satisfy one's appetite.

We should neither overeat nor eat less than what is required.

The yogis believe that one should fill half the stomach with food, a quarter with water and leave the rest empty for gases or air.

Meals should only be taken when one is hungry.

There should be a four-hour gap between the meals.

Water should not be taken with the meals. It could be taken half an hour before or after the meal.

The food should be chewed properly. Proper chewing of food helps in digestion and prevents overeating.

A good and balanced diet is the key to a sound body and mind.